# The Nurse Practitioner Survival Guide for New Grads

Catie Harris, PhD, AGACNP, FNP, ANP

ISBN: 0-9982519-7-6
ISBN-13: 978-0-9982519-7-4

## DEDICATION

To my son Matthew. My heart in everything I do.

# CONTENTS

# OVERVIEW

Nurse Practitioners (NP) have been around since 1965. Loretta Ford, widely regarding as the "mother" of NPs, forged the way for generations to follow her footsteps in providing advanced nursing care across the lifespan. Over 50 years of research has shown that NPs provide high quality care that is associated with excellent out- comes and lower cost. NPs have a masters or doctorate degrees in nursing which allows them to diagnose, treat and manage acute and chronic illness, as well as providing a focus on health promotion, wellness, disease prevention and patient education.

Opportunities for NPs have exploded in the last decade as the healthcare system has realized the important role we play in access and delivery of care to patients. When I started as a nurse practitioner in the early 2000s, our group had 2 NPs. Now we can't function with a group less than 15 NPs. This scenario is occurring all over the healthcare system. NPs are in demand and needed more than ever.

That first year of a new grad's life is tough! And there is a steep learning curve to master. I truly believe with help from this blue- print you can kick-start your own NP career and be successful.

This guide outlines the lessons I have learned over the years and the process I teach my own students right before they graduate from NP school. It is my hope that if you follow the steps in this guide you will be on a straight path to success in transitioning from the role of a nurse to a nurse practitioner over the next year.

Good Luck and Enjoy!

Catie Harris PhD, AGACNP, FNP, ANP
www.CatieHarris.com

# 1 INTRODUCTION

## Welcome

The first year of being a nurse practitioner (NP) is tough! Getting through graduate school, obtaining a license, certification and getting credentialed… there is a long list of things to be done! Then how do you know how to find a job, choose a specialty or interview?

Many new NPs take jobs for that may not be a good fit, but how do you know? Who is mentoring you through this process? In most cases you are on your own.

With the volume of nurse practitioner students graduating each term, finding a mentor to be invested in your career and your choices is getting harder and harder.

Everyone will undoubtedly survive their first year being an NP, but what if it could be easier, less stressful and more fun! Shouldn't that be the expectation, that somewhere, somehow, someone wrote a guide on what you need to do to be successful in your first year?

Well, welcome to the Nurse Practitioner Survival Guide for New Grads!

# Why I Wrote This Guide

So with the ongoing demand and rapid growth of the NP industry there are more new NPs coming out of University than ever before. This is a good thing because NPs are needed, but there is also a down side to having large quantities of a commodity produced – and that is sacrificing quality.

In my first couple of years teaching we had 8-10 acute care NP students graduate. In my last couple of years I have had 50-70 students graduating a year. As you can imagine in the smaller groups, I was able to coddle and nurture the students, walking them through the process of becoming an NP.

But now I am overwhelmed by the sheer number of assignments, paperwork and course load that I am required to teach to a large (and growing) number of students.

# What Happened To Preceptors?

This same scenario is occurring in clinical rotations as well. Preceptors are in demand more than ever and they are being asked to take up to a couple students at a time, semester after semester. What you experience is rapid burn-out. It becomes harder and harder to find a mentor or someone to really take a vested interest in your career.

New NPs are increasingly expected to step directly into the role of the NP, whereas we all know there is a transition period that is necessary for new grad NPs to function successfully. I have seen some new NPs do this gracefully and without a hitch, but they are few and far between. Most of us (myself included!) need someone to help navigate the role of the NP and understand our place.

# Why Create This Guide?

I created this guide to help the new NP to kick-start his/her own NP career. Nothing out there exists that is comparable to this guide. You can find all this information piecemeal, but it can take hours and you still don't know if you found everything you need.

This guide is intended to give you those hours back to relax and worry about other things. Go through the entire guide, complete the checklists and get ready to start your first job without worrying about what else you need to do.

# About The Author

Who am I? This is a good starting point to explain who I am and why I'm worth listening to! Let me start at the beginning and give you a bit of my journey.

I graduated from nursing school in the 90s and swore the two things I would never do were work on a neuro unit and work nights! But guess what, as fate would have it 1996 and 1997 were very bad years for new grads in nursing in the Philadelphia area, where I lived. There was such a surplus of nurses that hospitals who had paid nursing school tuition were turning away their own graduates.

It was a sad time in my life, having graduated college, living with my parents and working as an assistant trying to get a job. So I took a chance and applied for nursing jobs all over the United States and ended up in a tiny town in Texas called Victoria.

The caveat? I had to work on a neuro floor on the night shift! Ha! So much for absolutes… I would go on in my career to develop my love of neuro into many different projects (my dissertation), though I did get out of night shift after a couple years.

Three years later I went on for to obtain a master's in business administration (MBA) followed by my masters in Science for adult health NP. At the time, the adult NP degree was the most versatile, allowing me to work inpatient or outpatient. However, I would later regret this decision as I was forced to return for my post-masters in Acute and Family in order to work in the settings I wanted.

In 2011, I finished my dissertation after 6 long years and earned my PhD. During this time I built up my career as a nurse practitioner working in all aspects of neuroscience including inpatient, outpatient, neuro ED, neurotrauma, creating a comprehensive stroke center at a satellite hospital, first assist in the operating room and doing lectures and in-services around the country.

I built a really great niche around expertise in neuro. I created guidelines for all the nurses and providers in neuro to follow in my unit, which then led naturally to developing a neuro program. I created in-house neuro simulations and began recording lessons in how to become a neuroscience NP.

Finally, believing that our new NPs needed more guidance and mentoring, I created a neuroscience fellowship program that entailed achieving milestones in a structured manner. This allowed the new NPs to gauge where they were in the process and see if they were falling off track in any one area.

When my son was born, the long days, weekends and unpredictable hours (+ being on-call) of working with neurosurgery weren't practical for me, so I took a position at the University associated with my hospital as the director of the nurse practitioner program.

I really loved working in this position, which provided me with insights on the learning process of students. I wrote an **article** on the benefit and need of post-graduate residency programs and co-authored a qualitative study on the perceptions of readiness of nurse practitioner students at graduation.

**……then along came Walmart**

By 2015, Walmart had piloted its own version of retail healthcare in select stores in the South, specifically in Texas, South Carolina and Georgia. The model of using NPs to deliver primary care services in the retail setting was largely successful, so they began to build a team of NPs to scale the model and create the Walmart Care Clinics.

I got involved in this process through a friend of a friend who knew I knew a lot of people. Walmart was looking for an NP to lead Talent Acquisition and Professional Relations for the Walmart Care Clinics.

After hearing about the Walmart model and the job – basically to network with people and build the employment brand – I was so excited to join! Now in addition to my experience of

7

clinical work, project management, research and teaching, I have become an expert in recruiting and hiring NPs as well as branding and marketing concepts. I have a lot to teach and look forward to helping out as many NPs as I can.

So, I have had a lot of experience in this space. I know what new NPs need to start as nurse practitioners and I know what nurse practitioners need to achieve the next level in their careers.

Hopefully at this point, you also believe that I have the expertise to guide you through the process of becoming a nurse practitioner. I certainly look to your feedback as you move through this guide and any subsequent coaching you do with me, as learning is a constant iterative process.

# Why Doesn't Anything Like This Exist?

To date, I have not been able to find any online mentoring or coaching courses for new NPs despite the fact that more and more people are graduating.

There are a few post-graduate residency programs that exist across the U.S. to facilitate the transition from nurse to NP, however only a handful of new graduate NPs will be able to benefit from those programs.

More post-graduate residency programs aren't popping up, not because they aren't useful – on the contrary—these programs are great! However, they are very expensive and to date finding an entity to fund them has been very difficult.

**Post Grad NP Programs**
*not exhaustive, please google

Clin Hematolgy, VA
http://bit.ly/28IMR7A

Capital Health, NJ
http://bit.ly/1Up175h

Columbia ICU, NYC
http://bit.ly/1RXDRtl

Community FNP, Wash
http://bit.ly/28IM0Uz

Community FNP, CT
http://bit.ly/1Zztxxy

Emory, GA
http://bit.ly/1Up1bC1

Family NP, MA
http://bit.ly/218VDR0

John Hopkins GI/Hep, MD
http://bit.ly/1Up2lNW

Lahey Derm, MA
http://bit.ly/1swzRxr

MGH Pall Care, MA
http://bit.ly/1mx00ll

Mayo Clinic
http://mayocl.in/22RQ9eM

MD Anderson, TX
http://bit.ly/1tiQbAH

Memorial Sloan Kettering
http://bit.ly/1tiQbAH

St. Luke's Trauma, PA
http://bit.ly/22RR1QJ

UCSF, CA
http://bit.ly/1Pi8hXs

UMMS, MD
http://bit.ly/1UF988M

One post-graduate NP can cost a hospital or clinic over $100,000 to train in a structured program. If you are interested in a post-graduate residency program you should search for them. I encourage all my students to google the terms "post-graduate NP programs" or "NP fellowship" to find what is out there. Email and let me know if your own institution is starting something, so I can maintain an accurate database!

But what about the rest of us who can't move to Arizona or Minnesota to start a post-graduate residency program, no matter how great it is? What about those of us who can't take a big pay-cut in salary so that the program can be affordable to the institutions who host them?

What if you just want some structured guidance and coaching to help you through the first year and perhaps beyond?

As I said, I am not aware of anything like this that exists. Hence, I am writing this guide to provide structure to obtaining your first job because I believe in mentorship and guidance. I am hoping that this guide is a strong starting point for you. I would also encourage you to check out my website, CatieHarris.com.

The running theme throughout all the blog posts and podcast interviews is that no one did it alone. Everyone has a mentor of sorts who helped guide us through the process. I have had many mentors in the past, but rarely encountered the structure that I crave in learning until recently. I feel like I could be so much further along in my career if I could have understood the big picture earlier on.

So my goal in helping you is to move you along the continuum, to start you further up than where I started. Let's get your first job, let's choose your career trajectory, and let's map out the steps on how to get you there. After you complete this guide, consider the benefits you could gain from being coached and mentored from the start of your career. Well, the first step at this point is to graduate! And if you just graduated, let's get started with the first things you need to do.

# 2 READY TO GRADUATE

## Evaluate Your Situation

Presumably, if you are reading this you are either about to graduate or just newly graduated. Or maybe you are coming back to NP after a break. I know a lot of NP graduates who continued to work as a nurse for a couple years before taking on the role of the NP.

In any case, it's important to take a look at your own situation before you begin the process of becoming an NP or finding a job. Once job offers come rolling in you may be tempted to take a position that is not a good fit for you. The only way to know what a good fit means to you is to do an evaluation of yourself and your situation.

Let's start with a quiz. Don't leave yet! Not a typical academic quiz, this is all about you! Just choose the answer that most appeals to you, don't overthink it.

|  | Column A | Column B |
|---|---|---|
| What is your personality type? Choose the word you identify with at first glance | ○ Analyst or Diplomat* Architect, logician, commander, debater, advocate, mediator, protagonist, campaigner | ○ Sentinel or Explorer* Logistician, defender, executive, consul, virtuoso, adventurer, entrepreneur, entertainer |
| Do you prefer to work: | ○ In teams | ○ Solo |
| Do you like seeing: | ○ The whole picture | ○ Focus on a particular area |
| Are you more: | ○ Philosophical | ○ Results-oriented |
| Do you like focusing on: | ○ One thing at a time | ○ Multiple tasks simultaneously |
| Do you like coming to: | ○ The same environment | ○ An unpredictable location |
| Do you have | ○ Family or dependents | ○ No ties! |

*These personality types are based off the 16 dominant personality types as described by Myers-Briggs. To see a description of the various types, visit: http://bit.ly/1QYmkay

How did you do? What were your dominant predispositions? What does it all mean and what am I trying to get at?

# Quiz Results!

If you chose mostly in Column A you would probably be happier as a medical NP or working in an ICU setting, whereas Column B may mean you would enjoy being a surgical NP or working in an ED setting. Based on what rationale?

# I Have A Theory Of The "NP Personality"

This is by no means a real theory, but I have 20 years of experience I'm drawing upon. This theory came about after the 1000th student asked me which specialty would be best the best fit for them. I began to think about which qualities of the student seemed to fit best in which specialty.

So I looked to my own service to formulate some ideas. We had a bit of a transition where we separated out three types of patients, and our NPs essentially chose where they wanted to go. For example, the neurosurgeons wanted their own NPs, the neuro ICU attendings wanted their own NPs and the general neurology attendings wanted their own NPs.

# Different Facets Of NP Roles

So who went with whom?

The first level split I saw was whether the NP chose a medical service (Neurology), the surgical service (Neurosurgery) or the ICU.

This resonated with me on many levels. At the time, I had spent many years and many hours working long hours with neurosurgery. I wanted a service that was more predictable on hours, but still fast paced, so I chose the ICU. I loved working with the surgeons, but the hours were crazy. Neurosurgery tends to be fast-paced and narrowly focused (on the brain obviously). Neurosurgery patients in the ICU are also very challenging to work with and changes occur rapidly and unpredictably, but I had a relief at the end of the day to sign out to.

Medical NPs don't look at one specific organ such as the brain, they look at the whole person and deal with whatever issues present themselves. I see medical NPs like CSI investigators.

Medical NPs tend to own the issues to their best of their ability, whereas surgical NPs are taught to outsource any issue that is not related to the target organ. For example, as a neurosurgery NP, if my patient needs preop clearance, I would need to call the Medicine NP. Whereas a medical NP would care for the patient in the larger sense unless they needed something specific, like a surgical consult.

Medical NPs would also tend to round much longer on their patients because they do own the whole picture.

Neurosurgery rounds may last an hour, but we could literally "see" 45 patients in that time frame. This is the main reason we outsource most of our issues to medicine, because quite frankly you can't appropriately see 45 patients in an hour. But we can address just their main neuro issues that quickly as a team. A large part of your job as the Surgical NP on this team will be placing consults and following up on consults in between clinic, cases and discharges.

## ICU vs ED Personalities

The ICU fit with me because I like uncertainty of my day. There are days when nothing happens and days when everything seems to fall apart at the seams. I thrive on all of that.

The ICU may fluctuate in extremes of how sick the patients are and the types of crises that occur, but it's a relatively controlled setting. There is the physically limiting factor that there are only so many beds. Then there is the presence of many people and resources who can help you. Typically the physicians will park themselves on the unit when they have really sick patients, the nurses usually only have 2 patients and many people are involved in the case.

The fourth type of NP I categorize as an emergency department (ED) NP. I hate the ED. Why? While I just told you that I love the uncertainty of the Neuro ICU, it's still confined to neurosurgical patients. What I don't like about medical services and EDs is the general-ness of them. Let me break down what I mean about that a little bit more.

The ED will also fluctuate in extremes of how sick the patients are and how busy it gets, but the setting is not controlled at all. First you have no idea what is going to come through the door at any minute that you need to deal with.

Non-ED physicians and NPs hate to come to the ED. It is quite possible you might be on your own for long periods of time. Patients may quite literally be sprawled all over the place, in hallways, walking around, and in rooms you didn't realize existed.

I can't tolerate this level of chaos, but it is a huge appeal to some people.

So instead of thinking of which specialty per se you should work in, consider first what type of NP you are medical or surgical. Then consider if you are an ED or ICU personality. The ED personality likes unpredictable, uncontrolled chaos, whereas an ICU personality likes moderately unpredictable, yet controlled chaos.

## Inpatient vs Outpatient

The outpatient world is very different from the inpatient world. I'm not sure my theory can really extend as far as to provide assistance in choosing between these two settings. The role of the NP is continually evolving, but at the current time, most NPs regardless of certification can work in either setting. Since the LACE document came out, things are starting to change.

Although the LACE document clearly states that the populations are not Setting Specific, many institutions took a radical approach.

Credentialing boards in some major hospitals decided that only Acute Care NPs could work in the hospital. In order to see any patients in my hospital system, an NP needs to have the Acute Care NP certification, otherwise they will not get credentialed.

This is a case where Federal and State law allow us to practice, but local barriers change the rules. Anyway, almost 200 NPs in my hospital system had to go back and get the acute care certification in order to keep our jobs. Admission into the acute care NP program skyrocketed. However, once you leave the downtown area, most hospitals are still hiring Adult and Family NPs into the inpatient setting.

Conversely, acute care NPs can work in outpatient. So which should you choose? Again this is outside of my theory, however I can give you the pros and cons of each side.

| Outpatient | Pros | Cons |
|---|---|---|
| | Own panel of patients | Exposure to Insurance companies |
| | Very independent | Peer to Peer Reviews with Insurance Companies |
| | Coordinate care of your patients | Getting Tasked for everything |
| | Get great experience | Returning phone calls |
| | Learn entrepreneurial skills | Very fast pace, never ending list of things to do |
| | Learn healthcare system quickly | Getting auths, consults, approvals, tests done |
| | Office hours | Office hours |
| | Impact of NP care is obvious | Doing a lot of scut work and overflow from MD |
| | Oppty for billing/bonus | Having to bill for everything |
| | | |
| Inpatient | Work in groups | Minimal autonomy in a lot of places |
| | Get things done fast | Lacks exposure to how things operate |
| | Learn quickly | Rounding for hours |
| | Coordinated care of patients | Dealing with angry family members |
| | Working w/colleagues/consults | Chasing after consults |
| | No billing for most part | Very difficult to bill |
| | Interdisciplinary care | Interdisciplinary meetings |
| | | Being chased after by documentation specialists |
| | | Very difficult to show NP impact/worth |
| | | Usually no bonus since can't show worth |

The situation I liked the best was working both inpatient and outpatient neurosurgery. I did office hours on Monday, saw patients in the ICU, triaged neuro patients in the ED, scrubbed into the OR, did peer reviews during lunch with the Medical Director of the insurance companies, called patients back, etc.

When my situation changed, I found myself only in the ICU and I missed a huge part of the patient experience. When you only work inpatient, you don't understand the chaos of the outpatient world and vice versa, if you only work outpatient you don't understand the experience of missing information, screaming surgeons, cancelled OR, etc.

Outpatient NPs are generally much more independent. They are likely to have their own panel of patients and work independently. There is much more opportunity for negotiating salary in the outpatient world where the NP can show worth through billing charges. If you become a master biller, you could probably negotiate bonuses based on your performance.

Because inpatient NPs work in groups, the large majority of hospitals would bill under the physician's name. The NP will only get paid 80% of what the MD gets paid, so it would be like leaving 20% on the table. The down side to this scenario is the work of the NP is basically invisible.

What are you going to show as your contribution? Your contribution is intangible (and so will your bonus be!).

Ultimately if you get offered a job either inpatient or outpatient and you are not sure, shadow the NP for the day. Get a feel of what the job is like, particularly in the outpatient setting. Warning: It will be a whirlwind!

If you hate the in/outpatient setting after a year (give any job at least a year), then switch. There is no reason you can't move between inpatient and outpatient settings. Actually having the experience of both worlds makes you more valuable.

In Chapter 4 we talk more about getting a job, but ultimately, the most important aspect of any job is liking your colleagues and the atmosphere where you spend most of your day. Everything else should be secondary.

Now that we have assessed the type of person you are, let's keep that in mind and explore where your interests lay.

# Evaluate Your Interests

## The Types of NPs

What does that mean? I separate out the two types of NPs artificially, and that is not say one type of NP is superior over the other, they are just different avenues. Kind of like when you were a nurse, maybe you gravitated to the medical floor or maybe you were energized by the surgical floor. Maybe you liked ED or ICU.

Inherently, nurses self-select into a particular setting because it matches their personality or how they like to work.

It is the same thing as an NP. If you don't like working as a surgical nurse, you will likely not enjoy working as a surgical NP, so straight off the bat, you can narrow your focus to what you really want. Then when a position opens up in General Surgery for an NP, you know that is not the area you want and it may be worth waiting for something else.

And trust me unless you live in an area with one medical office and one hospital, opportunities will spring up. It's just like buying a house, great opportunities are always coming on and off the market. So don't settle too fast or too early.

Once you decide what your natural inclinations are, then you can decide what your interests are, first by ruling certain segments out. One of the most important parts of knowing what you want, is knowing what you don't want. Now the checklist above is not a hard-fast rule, it's a guide to help you understand who you are and where you will thrive.

Now let's think about your interests. I don't want you to narrow your interests down to a specialty quite yet. There may be specialties out there you don't know anything about but may be a good fit. So you don't want to limit yourself too much. The distinction between a surgical and a medical NP is a good enough start in narrowing your focus.

Here is a list of questions to ask yourself and reflect upon. Once you complete this, then we can continue onwards…

| Questions about yourself and goals | What was your original goal to become a nurse practitioner? |
|---|---|
| | What type of lifestyle do want for yourself? |
| | Where do you see yourself practicing? (geographic location; urban, suburban, rural?) |
| | What aspects of medicine do you find most appealing? |
| | Are there areas of medical practice (particular situations, types of patients, etc.) which you find difficulty in handling or make you uncomfortable? |
| | Which of your skills do you value highly and how do they intersect with your career choice? |
| Questions about practice characteristics in specialties | What is the level and style of patient contact (LT care, transitional care, consultative)? |
| | What is the lifestyle of the specialty (on-call, long days, unpredictable times) |
| | Is there a high turnover rate (i.e. burnout rate) in a particular specialty? |
| | What is the learning curve for a particular specialty (i.e. very steep for neuro ICU for NPs without ICU or neuro experience) |

So now you know who you are and where your interests lay, to get the right job at the right place. You will need to network a bit. More on that in the next chapter.

# Never Burn Your Bridges

Surely your parents or friends have told you not to burn your bridges. This could not be any better advice for anyone in the medical field. The fact of the matter is the

NP community is relatively small and we all talk to each other.

As the director of the acute care NP program I can tell you that each year I had to have a sit down talk with at least one student if not more to discuss their attitude at clinical.

For instance, the preceptors thought the student was bored or didn't care, the student would take 2 hour lunch breaks (not exaggerating), etc. When I would talk to the student, there was always

another side, but about half the time the student would admit to not liking the rotation, the preceptor wasn't interested in teaching, etc.. But guess what, when that student graduated, I can assure you they didn't get a job in the hospital where they did clinicals.

## The NP Community Is Small!

Why? Because, we all talk to each other. As soon as a newly graduated student applies for a job, my phone starts ringing. Who is this NP, were they good, where did they do clinicals, what did their preceptors say about them?

**Employers spend an enormous amount of money to recruit**
**and hire people into the company.**

One of the biggest measures for Human Resources is Quality of Hire. Basically, quality of hire is hiring a candidate who is a good match.

Unfortunately, objective data is not very helpful in judging quality of hire (after all it's a qualitative measure). A student with a 4.0 GPA is not necessarily the best NP for a service, just as the NP who graduated last in class isn't the worst. That isn't how it works. So the next best way to measure quality of hire is to get someone to vouch for your personality and fit.

## Your Reputation

*If you have a reputation in the hospital or office of being* **bored, lazy or uninterested** (even if it's not true to you), that perception will follow you.

What I tell my students and what I'm telling you know is you have to manage people's perception of you. This will not change through the course of your career – you will always have to manage it.

You have the power to change the way people see you. If you are sitting at the nurses' station playing on your phone and not participating then people will interpret this as bored and uninterested. If you spend your time constructing thoughtful questions and finding ways to be useful to the unit/service you will be viewed as enthusiastic and a team player.

Both these types of students may have the same academic performance, but the latter student will be in demand probably by multiple services. Trust me on this one, the NP community is small and mobile. Your preceptor today may be the next Chief Nursing Officer or maybe even one of your direct reports in a couple years. You never know, so do yourself a favor and don't burn bridges!!

# 3 GRADUATION

## Becoming A Nurse Practitioner

The process of becoming an NP is both physical and meta-physical. What do I mean by that before you shut me down?

Well there are the actual steps you take to get your NP license and certification, getting a job, being credentialed, etc. These are relatively easy and straightforward and what we will focus on next. The second part of becoming an NP non-tangible, such as thinking and acting like an NP, transitioning to a new role and working through the novice stages, which we will talk about a little later.

## First Steps

The very first step is to graduate from an accredited Masters program for Nurse Practitioners. The next step will depend on which state you are working in. Each state has its own rules and regulations regarding NP practice and who controls it. For most of the U.S., the individual state board of nursing monitors and regulates NP practice. Check out AANP map of state regulations: http://bit.ly/1MrEOHM

There are five (5) states where the state board of nursing AND the board of medicine regulate NP practice (Alabama, Florida, North Carolina, South Dakota and Virginia). In these 5 states, you may have additional requirements, so please check with your state nursing board regarding any additional steps you need to take (if any) to register with the board of medicine. There are also two (2) states that do not yet require national certification (California and New York).

If you are in either of these states, I would strongly recommend that you obtain national certification even if you think you will never step foot out of California or New York ever.

First, rules change, and in fact they can change dramatically very quickly. Given that California and New York are the only two states in the Union who don't require national certification, there is a high probability that it will change in the near future once enough pressure is applied by external agencies, i.e. other State Boards of Nursing, CMS, third party payors.

Second, it is much easier to take the boards when you are fresh out of school. Studies show the success of passing the boards is linearly related to the amount of time lapsed from the last class you took. Third, you may not be able to get credentialed by insurance companies without certification, which will severely limit your ability to negotiate your billing charges in the future. Finally, you cannot predict the future, so even if you don't think you will ever move, you still might, in which case you won't be able to practice in 48 other states.

# Licensure And Certification

Ok, so now you are ready to get licensed and certified, or certified and licensed. Back when I got my NP license in 2005, certification was optional, so I applied for my license first. But now the state boards of nursing want to see that you are certified to practice first.

So step number 1 is to get certified. But by whom? For Family and Adult (AGPCNPs) NPs there is certification available through AANP or ANCC. For acute care (AGACNP) there is ANCC or AACN.

What do I recommend? The real answer is – it doesn't matter. I am personally more familiar with ANCC. Since I am certified in three foci – adult, family and acute, I have that familiarity with ANCC, so my personal recommendation based on experience is just to take the certification exam with ANCC. ANCC is the only certification which handles adult, family and acute care.

AANP, according to my sources, has no intention of creating an acute care certification in the near future. I am not familiar at all with the American Association of Critical Care Nurses acute care certification course, however, in general I probably wouldn't recommend it.

Before the LACE document (http://bit.ly/1AI95mx), acute care really was just for ICU

NPs, so the certification exam through AACN probably made sense before 2008. Now, acute care refers basically to anyone in the hospital system, not just ICU.

So does it make sense to be a certified critical care NP? On the flip side of that question is, can a critical care NP exam be the basis for certifying all acute care NPs? There are too many questions and variables in the AACN exam for me, so my general advice for acute care NPs would be to take the ANCC exam and not worry about whether it will still be available in 10 years.

Regardless, go to the website of your choice and get moving on your application for national certification. You can start the application process several weeks to months in advance. Both ANCC and AANP will accept your credit card payment at any time! However, you will need

Step 1 – Get certified nationally!
Step 2 – Apply for licensure
Step 3 – Get credentialed by your facility
Step 4 – Get credentialed by insurance companies         (optional) Step 5
– Start working (finally!)

official transcripts sent in so they can verify you have indeed graduated from an NP program. For Family and Adult NP students, contact AANP (http://bit.ly/1YaEgjr)        or        ANCC (http://bit.ly/1ErEVPX) to get your application. For Acute Care NP students start at the ANCC website. ANCC also has certification exams for pediatric NPs, psychiatric NPs and emergency department NPs (AANP expects to have the ED certification out by 2017).

Be sure to celebrate the milestone of getting national certification. It's a huge weight off your shoulders. As soon as you figure out that you passed the boards, you can apply for your license – yes the same day!

And I would encourage you to apply for your license right away. You will need to go to your state board of nursing to figure out what is needed, but usually an application and more money. You will have the temporary national certification in hand, which can be used to verify you passed the boards. Applying to the state board will require a lot of the same documents you have already sent in to AANP or ANCC. No, they won't share information! So get it all out again.

Checklist for certification
- ⃝ Choose your certifying body (AANP or ANCC)
- ⃝ Start your application in the last semester of NP school
- ⃝ Make your credit card payment
- ⃝ Send in official transcripts (you need to pay for these to be sent, your school will not send them automatically. Make sure they don't get sent until you have officially graduated)
- ⃝ Your school of nursing will need to verify that you took pharmacology and did indeed graduate from that school.
- ⃝ Be sure to find out who is responsible for sending this information into ANCC or AANP!
- ⃝ Start studying; consider a review course and review books (doesn't matter which ones)
- ⃝ Approximately 6 weeks after your application is completely done you should get a window of opportunity to take the boards – typically 90 days
- ⃝ Take boards at the designated center
- ⃝ Hopefully pass! You find out immediately
- ⃝ If you don't pass on the first try, its ok, you will need to come up with a strategy plan to ensure you pass the next time
- ⃝ Now it's time for **step 2** to apply for an NP license!

# Collaborative Practice

Collaborative practice means you have an official document that is co-signed by a physician who will oversee your practice either directly or indirectly. Direct supervision requires the physician to be physically in the same space as you are. Indirect supervision may mean the physician will evaluate your care on a pre-determined basis. Some states require a monthly meeting, evaluation of 10% of your charts, sign offs or by NP request only.

Each state is a little different on what they require, so best to check out the website and go from there. Even states that have independent practice still may have some additional requirements.

For example, Alaska, which is an independent practice state still requires that NPs have a consultative and referral plan with an identified physician in order to practice; whereas in New Jersey, a reduced practice state, NPs only need to have a signed joint protocol in place with an identified physician. In Pennsylvania where I work, you need a collaborative agreement with a physician and a prescriptive authority license with two identified physicians.

If you require a collaborative practice agreement to be in place prior to working, chances are the facility where you are starting will already have something generic written out and ready for you to sign. If not, you can certainly use this template or borrow the joint protocol from the State of New Jersey Be sure to check you state board regulations to see if there are any absolute requirements of what should be included in the document.

Again keep a signed copy at all times on the cloud based share drive that I'm sure you just recently set up!

# Reciprocity

Once you have an NP license in one state, you can get a reciprocal license in another state. For instance, my NP license is in the state of PA. In order to obtain an NP license in NJ, I can claim reciprocity and of course pay the outrageous fees to the state board. This is in lieu of taking boards again.

Some states are RN compact, meaning if you live in state A and move to state B, you do not need a new RN license, you just need to apply for NP reciprocity. Unlike the state of NJ, where I needed to pay for an RN license first, then apply for NP reciprocity.

NP compact states are coming. In fact, Wyoming was the first state to join the NP compact, so hopefully in the near future, we can have one license for all states, (ahemm, California and New York excluded of course, since the bar to practice is not equivalent).

**Quick Tip:**
Keep a copy of all your documents in a cloud account such as Google drive, Dropbox or One Drive. You will be repeatedly asked for the same documents over and over. Best to keep them in one place where they can be easily and rapidly accessed.

# Titles

Now the tricky question. Once you are board certified and licensed as an NP, what initials do you use??

This is indeed a very tricky question. In the state of Pennsylvania, I am a CRNP, but in New Jersey I am an APN. However, my certification is AGACNP. In Florida, I would be an APRN.

The answer is – it depends.

If I am writing a medication prescription in the state of PA, I would use CRNP, since that is the state appointed designation for nurse practitioners. In NJ, I need to use APN.

If I am sending a resume to someone, particularly in a different state, I would use my national certification, so they could identify with my specialty, i.e. AGACNP.

You will notice on the front of this e-book, I use my national certifications. Why?

Because you as the reader may not have ever seen the designation CRNP before and you wouldn't know what it means. On the other hand, CRNP is for all NPs in Pennsylvania and it doesn't tell you if I'm a pediatric, family, adult, psych, neonatal NP, etc.

You will need to figure out what the proper title for writing prescriptions and signing official documents is in your state. Then I would reserve your board certification acronyms for anything to do with your career, i.e. getting a job, giving presentations, writing papers, etc.

# 4 FINDING A JOB

Finding an NP job is not really the hard part. What is tough is finding a job that you want as well as finding a job that will mentor you as a new nurse practitioner.

With increasing demands for NPs continue to escalate, the expectation is that new grads are coming out practice-ready. When I first graduated my service knew they wanted an NP but weren't quite sure what to do with me. I flew under the radar for a while doing my own thing.

This was both good and bad. Good, because it gave me the chance to learn about the role of the nurse practitioner and ease into it, taking things at my speed.

**It was bad because I spent a year dilly-dallying at my new job when I should have been making strides at launching my career.**

I hadn't learned much about the specialty because there were no expectations of me. Nowadays, the complete opposite is true. The new grads we hire onto my service are expected to function at a high level pretty quickly.

It's great that the bar is set high for NPs, but there has to be some mechanism in between to help facilitate not only the role transition, but the support the knowledge deficit. We lost many NPs over the years because they couldn't "get" neuro.

But the fact of the matter is, the service didn't "get" how to mentor the NPs into the role.

# Choosing A Specialty

To get your first job, do you choose a specialty or do you let the specialty choose you? I've had students over the years who wanted to do 3 and 4 rotations per semester so they could get exposure to the different specialties.

**Quick Tip:**
First go back and decide if you are a medical NP or surgical NP. Then you can let the specialty opportunities choose you.

The most I've ever let any student do is 2 specialties in one rotation. Medical students spend their last two years in school rotating on and off various services and for good reason.

Once a medical student declares a specialty in medicine, they are basically stuck in that field. At the very least it's very difficult and expensive to change specialties. If a medical student decides dermatology is the specialty she will go into, then they have to match to a program, do residency for several years and then likely do some sort of sub-specialty training. If that same student decides she doesn't like dermatology after graduation and wants to be a general surgeon, guess what it will be very hard to change course.

Not so with the NP role. You can certainly spend years learning a specialty role and I would encourage you to do that. But if you start in the ICU and 5 years into it you decide you would rather work in a dermatology office you can change with relative ease.

The hardest part about making the switch is finding a practice that is willing to train you. At this point most places are very open to training. So let's say choosing a specialty is not a make or break proposition. As we talked about before, I would predetermine if you are a medical NP or a surgical NP first. Then I would do a combination of looking for jobs in an area you think you would like, but remain open to everything.

For example, if I decide I'm a medical NP and I want to work in a high energy setting such as the ICU, does it really matter if I work in the medical ICU, the Burn unit, the CCU or the Neuro ICU.

Not really. All these specialties are going to have a steep learning curve, and they will likely function in a similar manner.

The difference among them is the knowledge content. Will you focus your energy on deep learning of the function of the heart or the brain or the skin or general medical issues? In this case, I would let the specialty choose you.

More important than the actual specialty is the group that works in the specialty. We will talk about interviewing later in this chapter, but what the unit is like is 1000x more important than which organ you learn about.

Now if you decide you are a surgical NP, you will also want to consider if there is an opportunity to first assist in the operating room as well.

You will want to know this up front. Some surgical practices just want the NPs to do the pre-op clearance and post op checks in the office and/or in the hospital.

Some surgical services expect the NPs to cover the OR on days when the residents are in classes or clinic. If you work in a community hospital there may be an expectation that you are in the OR whenever the surgeon is. It is best to know up front and will be part of your due- diligence in researching each job you apply for.

However, before you can apply for a job, you need to dig out a resume or CV

## Resume Or CV

What is the difference between a resume and a CV? They are pretty much used interchangeably these days, but technically a CV is a snapshot of your life's work, whereas a resume is a summary of your experience. I wouldn't get hung up on it.

If a place of employment asks for either a CV or a resume, you will send the same document. We will stick with the term 'resume' for the sake of this e-book.

There is a misconception that your resume must only be 1 page in length.

In my position of Senior Manager for Talent Acquisition I can tell you I have literally reviewed hundreds of resumes. The length itself does not matter to me in the least.

In the order of importance (and these are the things that should stand out)

I want to know what type of NP you are – Family, Adult, Acute, Psych, Neonatal, Peds, Women's Health.

I want to know what your experience is to date

We talked earlier about title designation. I get very frustrated when NPs put just CRNP, APN or APRN after their names and then never indicate which NP track they completed. It matters!

Make sure it is obvious on your resume which NP track you completed, preferably in your initials. For certain positions, I can only hire Family NPs because of the pediatric portion of their training. So I will sort through all the resumes I have to find resumes of FNPs. If it's not clear, the other resumes go into a pile that I may or may not revisit depending on whether or not I find a decent candidate in the first group. It's no good if you are an FNP, but your resume says:

Jane Doe, APN, University of the World

Masters of Science in Nursing 20XX

How will I know if you are qualified or not for the position, it would take some work to

figure it out. The one thing you don't want to do is make the recruiter or hiring manager work at figuring out whether or not you are qualified. Make it easy!! Now consider these two headings instead (both acceptable):

Jane Doe APN,

University of the World, 20XX

Masters of Science in Nursing – Family NP track

OR

Jane Doe, FNP

University of the World, 20XX Masters of Science in Nursing

The second most important part of your resume is your experience.

More years of experience as an RN does not necessarily make you a better NP. Showing increasing roles and responsibilities as an RN does!

How many years were you an RN and what were those years of experience like? An RN with 4 years of experience on a medical unit with charge responsibilities is much more compelling to me than an RN with 10 years of experience in an ICU.

Why? Because there is the general rule of diminishing returns. An RN with more years of experience doesn't give that person a greater edge to becoming an NP If anything, it may be harder to train someone who has been doing the same thing for so long. Then I start wondering why a RN whose has worked for a decade in the same place bothered to go to NP school, maybe they were burnt out on the unit and thought it would be easier to be an

NP? Fair? Maybe not, but it's my thought process. This is the kind of bias you need to watch out for when crafting your resume.

Make sure you highlight aspects of your RN career that were important, such as being charge nurse, doing staffing, heading up committees, winning unit awards, etc. Let's take a scenario and see how we can spin it into a positive resume entry.

RN with 2 years of experience but no evidence of increasing responsibility

- Provide a description of your home unit

- Focus on your clinical rotations, list them out and add references

- If you have no evidence of responsibility, go into work and join a committee, then put it on your resume. It's important to show involvement. You will be a better person and your unit will appreciate the extra hand as well.

**Example Resume:**

Registered Nurse Progressive Care Unit
World Hospital System, 5/20XX – Present
Progressive care nurse, skilled in the management of acute stroke and cardiac patients. Focused on evidence based practice, patient advocacy and transitions of care
> Experienced in providing nursing care to adult and geriatric populations with a variety of complex medical conditions including cardiology, oncology, surgical, acute exacerbation of multiple chronic co-morbidities and end of life care

> Member of various committees including Unit Council and the World Hospital Nursing Policy and Procedures Committee

> Nurse Practitioner Student Clinical Rotations Neurosurgery Service Fall, 20XX

> World Hospital, Philadelphia, PA Preceptor: Jane Doe, CRNP Managed pre and post-surgical patients in the hospital and outpatient setting.

> > Completed HPI and physical examinations for adolescent, adult and gerontology patients.
> > Presented patients and plan of care to attending surgeon on daily rounds.
> > Ordered and evaluated imaging and laboratory tests.
> > Ordered medications and consults.
> > o Discharge planning and follow up appointments.

Palliative Care Consult Service  Spring, 20XX

World Hospital, Paoli, PA Preceptor:  Cynthia Smith, CRNP

Clinical rotation in Palliative Care and Pain Management service, focused on the evaluation and management of acute and chronic symptoms such as pain, dyspnea, nausea, anxiety, delirium, and end-of-life care.

Provided psychosocial, counseling, and spiritual care to patients and families within an interdisciplinary team setting.

Participated in Palliative Care consultations. Gathered relevant information from medical record and reported to team.

Internal Medicine - Critical Care Summer, 20XX
World Hospital, Paoli, PA Preceptor: Jen Jones, CRNP

Managing a variety of medical, surgical and trauma patients in a 16 bed ICU.
Completed HPI and physical assessments on adult and

gerontology patients. Presented patients and plans to attending physicians on daily rounds.
Ordered and evaluated diagnostic imaging, laboratory, and serological tests.
Ordered medications and consults.
Responded as part of code team to all code blue and rapid responses in the hospital.

Not only is this a great resume from an NP with little RN experience and NO NP experience, but we hired her on our neurosurgical service. The resume was clean, professional looking and it seemed like she had lots of good rotational experience in clinicals.

By naming her preceptor, we got the impression that she felt confident they would say good things about her as well if we were to call them up. And remember what I said about the NP community being small.

Guess what? I knew these preceptors and did call them up. My group initially didn't want to hire this individual because she had no NP experience, but her preceptors thought so highly of her I was able to change my team's mind. Remember not to burn your bridges!

If you decide later on you want to work with me in building out your career trajectory in my course: The New NP Mentoring Program, we will build the foundation to transform your resume into a CV and figure out the most important areas to concentrate on to get to point B.

Everything else on your resume will be necessary fluff as far as I am concerned. Make it clean, easy on the eyes to scan and hit these key points:

1. Which NP track did you complete?

2. How many years of RN experience do you have

    a.   What evidence do you have of increasing responsibility

    b.   Which clinical rotations did you do and what skills did you acquire

3. Remember to put preceptors names provided you didn't burn bridges

Now that we have the resume pulled together let's talk about how to hunt down a job.

# Job Hunting

Once you have your resume pulled together, start sending it out. But to where??? In acute care this is probably more straightforward. Go to the hospital where you want to work and look at the job postings in their career site.

For positions in offices, it's not always so easy. Smaller office practices may rely more on word of mouth and networking because they may not even have a website, let alone a career board. So let's go over a couple options of places you can go to hunt down jobs – and you may need to be creative!

Several years ago, I was so frustrated that our HR department was so slow in posting a position that we desperately needed filled. It had been almost 2 months and the job wasn't even posted. I took it upon myself to post the position on Craigslist on the internet.

And guess what within a week, we had two applicants, two interviews and one new hire. Now how was that for service! Did it occur to you to go onto a place like Craigslist? In retrospect, Craigslist was probably not the best avenue for a professional job search to be undertaken, but it was clearly effective. But it does highlight the power of communicating where people are talking or looking.

# Leveraging Social Media

You can do an internet search for the position you want or just google "nurse practitioner" jobs, but you will need to weed through a lot of unrelated information.

My suggestion would be to place your resume on a job board such as Indeed, Simply Hired, Glassdoor, etc. There are literally hundreds if not thousands of recruiters who are actively searching the resume banks for this information.

**Quick Tip:**
Put your resume on:
* Glassdoor
* Simply Hired
* Linked In
* HealthCareers
* ENP Network

As the Senior Manager for Talent Acquisition, I can tell you we spend a very large amount of money to access to all the job boards for nurse practitioners, as does every other large employer. We also buy resumes from the state and national organizations.

It is free for you, so why not just post your resume and let people beat down your door instead of looking? You can also use these job boards to search for jobs as well.

I am on Glassdoor and every week I get a list of all the open jobs that have been posted related to nurse practitioners. I am personally just interested to know what is out there! Some of the positions are things I would never have thought of to apply to. Many insurance companies want and use nurse practitioners or retail healthcare.

There are so many opportunities it can be just overwhelming.

The next place we spend a lot of money on is paying for a recruiter license on Linked In.

What???

You thought Linked In was just for business people? Guess what, half my list are other recruiters searching for nurse practitioners who aren't really on Linked In (because they think it's just for business people).

Again, Linked In is free and you should be on there! If you put yourself down as a nurse practitioner, I promise you that you will get a ton of unsolicited in-mails to respond to recruiters looking to place you in your dream job. It may even get to the point where you need to stop checking your messages.

Be sure to upload a picture on Linked-In. Don't be one of those persons with a ghost photo

Put a little effort into your profile so that you can be found.

- Headline – add some keywords that represent you, for instance be sure to mention that you a nurse practitioner (and use your national certification credentials!)

- Do Post a nice professional picture – go to the effort, to have one decent picture taken, it doesn't have to be professionally done, just follow these DON'T guidelines
  - o Do NOT post the ghost picture
  - o Do NOT post a picture of you in a group
  - o Do NOT post a picture of you in unprofessional situations
  - o Do NOT post a picture of you with the person next to you cropped out.

- Summary – this is 2000 character max. If you aren't sure what to write, look at other people's profiles for some suggestions

- Jobs – use standards titles so other people will know what you are talking about. For instance if you are a Senior Resource Nurse – I just made that up, but I don't know what it means. Instead just write:
  - o Registered Nurse – Responsible for championing nursing excellence for a 25 bed ICU as a resource expert

- Multimedia – Be sure to link your other social media files here, or a website or even any documents you want to share

- Groups – Finally there is a function called Groups. You can have up to 50 groups to help you network and meet other people. Join some nursing groups and build your network.

The last place I think most people think of, but is certainly the way of the future is looking for jobs on Facebook.

More and more companies are getting savvy to direct and indirect job advertisements on Facebook. They are finding different ways to get your attention and will continue to seep into Facebook. Hey there are over 1 billion users of Facebook and the advertising is dirt cheap!

## Networking for a job cannot be overstated.

This is how I came across my job as Senior Manager. A friend of a friend of mine told me that the Walmart Care Clinics were looking for a nurse practitioner. This amazing opportunity just literally fell in my lap and it's been the most exciting experience.

You can network online, offline, it doesn't matter. You just need to communicate to people that you are looking for a position. People come out of the woodwork for nurse practitioners.

The only caveat I would put here is that it can sometimes be tough to land that very first job. Many employers may be overwhelmed at the prospect of hiring a new grad, so definitely throw some thought into beefing up your RN experience, because that will sell more than anything. Once you have 1 years of experience, basically the world is your oyster! Enjoy!!

Things you should do to network:

- Talk to people and let them know you are looking for an NP job

- Post your resume on a job board and review the openings posted

- Search open positions in places where you want to work

- Set up a professional looking Linked In account and identify as a nurse practitioner

- Don't shy away from recruiters, they know everything about the market – talk to them

# Interview Tips

Now you have a rocking resume, you have done your job search and now you are getting ready to interview for a job that you think looks awesome.

Take a deep breath!

Remember job hunting is a lot like house hunting. You may find a job that appears to be everything you ever wanted and is the only one for you, but you have to control your emotions in making important decisions.

If you went step by step through this guide, hopefully you only lined up interviews for positions that match your NP personality.

Remember there are a million amazing jobs (and houses) out there that will fit with your lifestyle, finances and personality. The key is to understand they may not be there the second you begin to look for a job. It may be several months before the right job comes along, so be patient and don't settle just to get experience.

The first year is really hard and the wrong place can break your spirit and damage your self-confidence. I have created an online mentoring program to help new grads in that transition role that I encourage you to check out – The New NP Mentoring Program.

# How To Prepare

How do you prepare for an interview? Honestly, I would research the institution you are going to or the office. Know who is in charge, maybe search out/google some information about the hospital/office. However, at this stage I would not spend a whole lot of time on this. You are most likely not going to be grilled about who the CEO is and do you know what the P&L looks like on the hospital's financials.

I have been through 8 hour interviews where I just go from person to person finding out about who they are and what they do. Half the time the person isn't really expecting you, but stops for 10 minutes to "chat".

This "chat" with you may seem benign, but it is the critical aspect of your interview. Every person you interview with is going to send feedback into HR about whether or not they should hire you.

What is it based off of? Largely your personality. Most places want to know if you are going to be a cultural fit. And the interviewers are human, presumably without much HR training. There is no standardized method for hiring nurse practitioners that is validated for hiring managers. Interviews are almost a purely qualitative evaluation.

Some places will do behavioral interviews, which will judge you on your responses to situations, but it's very hard to prepare for the scenarios. The night before the interview, it might help to reflect on your nursing career and jot down some situations where you acted like a leader, helped out a peer, dealt with a difficult situation/patient/family, and managed others (such as a charge nurse, or how you led your NP student group, etc)

Make sure as you understand the "informal" interview as you are going through the motions. Remember, they want to know that you will fit in. You need to take your cue from this as well. In these "chats" you have throughout the day, you should be evaluating them and making notes of your feedback (to yourself).  When each person spoke to you:


- Were they frazzled and unorganized (this is probably good insight on a typical day)

- This is ok if you are not going to report directly to this person, but not ok if it's the Lead NP, it's a sign of the work environment

- Were they fun to talk to? This is important, because you will be working with them

- Did they speak badly of others? Trust me they will do the same to you if you work there. I can't tell you how many times on interviews the head of the department made disparaging remarks about the NPs or admins or whomever.  Bad sign!!

- Does the person showing you around talk to others? If they ignore everyone, it's probably because they don't have a collegial relationship


You have to look at the interview process as a time to see if you will be a cultural fit in that environment. Don't get hung up on whether or not you will get the job.


More often than not, we have taken candidates who just seemed to fit in the organization. We use their credentials or experience to upsell or downsell our own interactions.


For instance, in discussions of candidates, we took one person because they had no NP experience – apparently it would easier to mold her. But we didn't take another candidate because they had no NP experience. We do the reverse as well. We took one candidate because she had a ton of neurosurgery experience, but in another candidate that was seen as a negative and a reason not to hire. It would have been too hard to un-train and retrain her.

## Hiring Manager Selection

In dealing with my hiring managers, I see a lot of the same methodology. One hiring manager seems to only hire NPs with a bubbly personality and the other only likes the more serious type of interviewee.

No matter how much you think you want a particular position, the most important part of any job interview is figuring out if you would like to be there and if they would like to have you. This is a win-win scenario.

You don't want to be desperate and take a job out of haste and conversely you don't want a job that is equally desperate to have you (bad sign!!). So be very thoughtful in choosing your interviews. Don't turn down interviews because you want palliative care, but the Neuro ICU calls you instead to interview. It's worth seeing what the position is and who the people are, because as I have said before, your work environment is much more important than your work specialty.

Finally, do not bring up salary during your initial interview. Unless the employer brings it up, the interview is not the right time and it's in bad taste. For hospitals in particular, salary is negotiated with Human Resources.

The NP on the unit has absolutely no say in what you get paid. Don't ask for a range or ask the NPs how much you should expect. This is the one area that you should do your homework in. Check out min-max and average salaries for your geographic area and then by NP track. This will give you the ballpark area.

**Asking about salary at an interview will just leave a bad taste in everyone's mouth.**

More on salary and contracts in the next section.

# Negotiating A Contract

The most burning question as a new grad NP you will have about a job is how much money will you make? This is an excellent question and one that could make or break a potential job opportunity. So why don't they just tell you up front? Well for one, it's competitive information.

Most organizations guard those numbers so they have a little leverage for negotiating in case you have other opportunities.

Below are recent numbers for experienced NPs, so you should expect less for the most part, but it will also depend on where you live.

| | 2014 | 2013 | 2012 |
|---|---|---|---|
| Average FT Salary | $103,000 | $98,000 | $93,000 |

I am going to tell you straight out that in general for new graduate NPs, there is very little wiggle room in the salary negotiations. I have heard of new grad NPs walking away from jobs because of a $0.50 difference or for $1 an hour.

Do you know what that works out to be? Let's say Hospital A offers $44 per hour, but you wanted a minimum of $45 per hour. Is it worth losing an opportunity over? Well $44/hour amounts to an annual salary of $91,520 and $45/hr equals $93,600 or a difference of $2080. If you break it down a little more, that is $173 a workday or $0.75 per workday.

For a first job, is this really worth fighting over? The HR department has certain bandwidths they cannot go past without explicit approval from the hiring manager. If it gets to that level of negotiating and the hiring manager agrees, then you win right?

Well, guess what, maybe not. There may be a much higher expectation that you are practice ready. Since you get paid more than other new grads, the expectation will be you perform exponentially better to warrant the time and effort you made everyone go through to get the extra $1 that you likely would get within a year anyway.

I'm by no means saying do not negotiate your salary, because more often than not the HR department will give you the middle of the bandwidth salary.

What I am saying is that it is not worth negotiating a salary as a new grad that requires management intervention. Now if the salary you were expecting is nowhere even near the bandwidth that you are given, then you need to look for another job.

Let's say you know you can get $90k at any hospital, but you are offered $80k then you have to be willing to look elsewhere. It's not worth the effort to negotiate because nothing will make up the difference.

# Extra Benefits

There are other benefits that are more valuable than an extra $0.50/ hour. Consider asking the hospital to pay for your licenses, prescriptive authority license (in applicable states), DEA number – this just cost me $731 out of pocket to renew. Also make sure you get time off for continuing education, conferences and allowance for attending webinars, seminars and other educational endeavors. Your continuing education allowance should be at least $1500.

It is very hard to attend even one conference for less than that. And at the very least you should be attending one conference a year – preferably AANP as a new grad, but also your specialty organization conference. If your hospital doesn't value this, then you might also want to reconsider the job at this point as well. Does the hospital pay for you to belong to your specialty organization or to AANP? Will they pay for subscriptions to journals? All these benefits need to be considered when you are offered a job.

If your income is based off RVUs (relative work units) or billing productivity, this may be another avenue of negotiation. For a new grad NP you can expect that you are going to be much slower than a seasoned NP, so you wouldn't want your salary to be dependent on how many billable hours you have.

Make sure you know this up front. But you may want a productivity bonus once you are very skilled. Ask what kind of bonus structure they have. This may not be applicable in services where NPs do not bill.

Knowing who pays for your salary, i.e. where does the money come from, is important though if you are going to negotiate at any point in your career.

So in conclusion, don't ask about salary on an interview — it's like asking for a kiss before you finish dinner on a first date. Just let it happen.

When the offer does come up through HR, definitely ask for more as you see fit. Make sure you do your homework and know the expected ballpark salary you should be expecting.

Don't go into a place and demand $150k, this is not market value for a new grad NP by any stretch of the imagination. HR will let you know when they can't go any further and you need to decide at that point if you want to take the job or not.

Don't make your new manager go to bat for you this early in the game. When you have experience as an NP, you will potentially have skills worth negotiating for, but as a new grad, you are pretty much the same as any other candidate. Ask for extra benefits instead, this will make you look like a superstar and motivated NP.

# Non-Compete

One caveat, I have heard of some hospitals or offices requiring you to sign a non-compete. I would strongly advise you not to continue in the hiring process with an institution that wants a non-compete. Usually a non-compete clause has a radius, such as you wouldn't be able to work in any location within a 20-mile radius of that institution.

First, it can be devastating to you if the position doesn't work out, you essentially have to move or tolerate a very long commute somewhere else.

Second, it's a huge red flag. If the only way an institution can keep its NPs on board is by preventing them from working elsewhere nearby, not good!

Hopefully you would have seen these red flags when you interviewed the institution. The non-compete clause should cement your decision not to work there!

# Credentialing

Finally, you graduated, discovered your NP personality, applied for a job, interviewed and got the salary you wanted! Now you can start working right? Well, not really.

What is the credentialing process? The Medical Staff Affairs (MSA) office of any hospital system regulates the quality and assurance of credentials of any provider who wants to operate in that facility.

For example, for physicians and nurse practitioners, the MSA will require a very large application to be completed. It will look very much like the application that you filled out during the interview process.

Rest assured, you will need to do it all over again. In retail healthcare or smaller offices, this may just be the medical director in conjunction with an office manager who assumes this function. Essentially, credentialing is about making sure you have the proper credentials at all time. How formal and complicated the process is will be determined by the individual hospital or office.

The credentialing application will ask you about where you went to school followed by asking you questions of your competency in various tasks and skills. The MSA office will also verify and keep a list of your credentials, certifications, licenses and skills. You will need to supply your BLS, ACLS, Licenses, maybe even your graduate diploma. You will need to acknowledge that you understand the policies of the hospital system and that you have completed HIPPA training, etc.

Each hospital system is different, but most places will not let you start working or even orienting until you are credentialed by the MSA. It has been my experience that the MSA office at most places only meets once a month. So if you don't get your application in to the office in a timely fashion you could be waiting weeks before you can start.

My own horror story with the credentialing office at one hospital system was that each month they met and reviewed my file, there was some new missing item. This meant each month, I had to resubmit the application with the missing item.

In addition, the hospital had issues verifying my license with the State Board of Nursing for some crazy unknown reason.

Ultimately, from the day I was offered the job until I was credentialed and able to start working = 6 months.

Come to find out, it was a chronic problem at this hospital. Fortunately it was a second job for me, so I wasn't stressed out about it. However, I meant another guy who lived off credit cards until the credentialing committee finally came through about 6 months later for him as well.

Scary!! Don't quit your RN job until you have a start date!!!

Again, my suggestion to you is to have a copy of all your licenses, diplomas, certifications, skills, continuing education credits, ppd verification, etc. on some type of cloud based system, where you can just print them wherever you may be.

You don't want to waste time looking for those documents. I can assure you, you will need to produce them over and over again during the course of your career. In fact, once you are done getting credentialed with the hospital or office, you will need to do it again for all the insurance companies!

**Do yourself this huge favor and get organized.**

# 5 ROLE TRANSITION

## First Days On The Job

There is no way you have gone through a bachelor and master's degree in nursing and not know who Pat Benner is or her famous Novice to Expert model. Benner literally transcends nursing because her model is applicable to just about any situation where you go from your comfort zone to a new role. Just in case you were living under a rock and are somehow not familiar with this concept, let me walk you through it – it's important to understand!

## Novice To Expert

In the novice stage the learner has no experience with situations in which they are challenged to perform tasks. Novices need structure and rules to facilitate achievement of the first milestone. The novice stage is not the time to present theoretical speculations on why a medication or treatment may or may not work.

It is important to provide algorithms of care which provide the scaffolding of the knowledge base. At this level, the information provided to a novice should be dogma. As the new NP advances, it will be important to teach the novice to challenge the dogma, but not now. Because medical care is never the same for every patient every time, the novice needs to work with an NP preceptor who provides hard fast rules, but who is competent enough to know when the rules need to be adjusted or altered.

Without solid structure, the shear amount of incoming information can be so overwhelming the new NP could shut down. If this happens to you, you need to stop, reset and start at point where you are comfortable again.

If you have not started in your role as an NP yet, you can expect to start at this novice level. There is no set timeframe to say how long you will be there. Some NPs may advance rather quickly through this stage, but a lot of you won't. You will probably remain in this stage for about 6-12 weeks.

In the advanced beginner stage the learner starts to gain experience and starts to see meaningful patterns. The advanced beginner may start to recognize the times when the hard-fast rules learned in the previous stage don't apply.

There should be a shift in learning from hard fast rules to guidelines The advanced beginner may struggle with prioritizing issues and identifying important aspects of patient care. Once the advanced beginner is off orientation, ongoing mentoring is essential. It would be wise to pair up the advanced beginner with a competent NP for up to 1 year. This competent NP should be available for curbside consults whenever the advanced beginner is on the job. It may be helpful to a couple people for the learner to be able to call for help.

In the competent stage, the new NP is much less afraid to go to work!

A competent NP knows what s/he knows and knows what s/he doesn't. The competent NP can distinguish between relevant and irrelevant attributes, is able to cope and manage unforeseen events and starts using evidenced based practices to make decisions.

A note of warning, many people stop at this level. It's a tough, long road to reach competency as an NP in your specialty. Once you do, you may feel a certain level of comfort and weight lifted. Do not be fooled into staying at this level. If you have any unrealized dreams and aspirations for your career, even if it's just a spark or general sense of being, this is the time you need to work the hardest.

You will have just enough knowledge at this point to be good and not dangerous, but not enough to be remarkable or even stand out among your peers. You will just be one of the NPs on the unit or in the office. This stage starts usually at the 1 year mark, though as I said, you may be sooner or later than that anniversary. It's like a baby, some babies walk at 9 months, some walk at 15 months, it's all good.

The competent stage can last from year 1 to infinity if you let it. But I encourage you, do not get stuck in this stage. The hardest part is yet to come, but you will get the most rewards by pushing onwards.

If you choose to go onto the proficient stage, you will find you can synthesize complex case studies rapidly and hone in on accurate elements of problems with relative ease. You will see situations as a whole, rather than pieces of a whole.

This will take deliberate effort on your part to develop your knowledge base and to expand your scope of skills. Ironically, when you first start orientation, most employers will send you on a whirlwind tour of other services. I find this disorienting and overwhelming. New NPs do not need to be exposed to 5 or 6 different services while they are trying to learn 1 specific service.

Conversely, proficient NPs would benefit immensely from being exposed to other services and learning new information. At this level, you may need to take the initiative to make those experiences occur.

At the proficient level, you will be expected to navigate your own course to becoming an expert. Many people are not able to do this and can also get stuck in this proficient stage. The other fallacy is that some proficient NPs think they are experts but they are lacking some crucial attributes.

The expert NP is nothing less than a national treasure! The expert NP is a subject matter expert who is recognized as such by others. The expert NP grasps situations intuitively and correctly without wasting time. The expert NP can manage clinical problems in a fraction of the time it takes anyone else and provides excellent, exemplar care.

# Expectations

What are the expectations on the first day of your job? Well the bar starts out pretty low. If you start out with a fll panel of patients and no orientation – you should reconsider this job. Remember you have a license to protect!

On the first day of orientation, you are basically shown the lunch room, where you will work, you will meet some of your co-workers and probably shadow someone. Basically, it's like a week of Simon-says.

Your preceptor gets up, you get up, your preceptor sits down, you sit down. Though please allow the preceptor some privacy when going on bathroom breaks!

After the first two weeks of shadowing or learning about your facility and computer system, there will be some expectation that you start interacting with patients and performing some semblance of your job. You shouldn't be seeing patients on your own, your preceptor should see and sign off on every person you touch.

Remember, the Novice to Expert model. You will need some hard, fast rules. It may be a good idea to peruse the policy and procedures manual (this may be the only time ever that you look at them).

**I would also carry around a notebook to write down all useful numbers, code combinations and procedures for doing things.**

I used to have a phone notebook, so if I wrote down how to use the phone or make long distance calls, those instructions would go under P (for phone). If I needed to remember how to access the lunchroom code or nursing locker room, I would put both those under C (for Codes). If you are really obsessive, you can have a directory in the back of your book of the different words you use, but this might really be too much effort on this one thing!

Most orientations will last about 12 weeks. Some will be longer, but they should not be much shorter. The worst reason to take you off orientation is because the facility is understaffed. Being off orientation should not have anything to do with staffing and everything to do with your competency level.

You are not the best judge of your own competency. Most new NPs never believe they are ready to come off orientation. You get comfortable under the support of your preceptor.

However, you may feel like you aren't learning as much as you think you should. This may not be anything you have done or not done. It may be a preceptor issue that is the problem.

The proficient and expert NPs are frequently called upon to mentor new grad NPs in the beginning stages, however this may not always be the best scenario. Proficient and expert NPs may have a hard time using rules to teach.

**To the new NP it may seem like the answer to everything is: "it depends".**

This can be overwhelming and the new NP may shut down believing the learning curve is too steep. On the other hand the proficient and expert NPs may have trouble deconstructing their thought process. Proficient and expert NPs may lack the ability to recapture the mental processes required to make decisions in order to explain it to the novice NP.

Therefore, if you are orienting with a proficient or expert NP and feel like you aren't learning like you should, there may be a very logical explanation for this. And the answer may be to get an NP who isn't so far ahead of where you are in your education process to show you the rules and the ropes. Consider asking for a different preceptor for some time to see if it makes a difference. I wouldn't suggest making a production out of the request.

If you think your preceptor is too "expert" to teach, just innocently ask if you can follow NP Smith or whomever for a few days. You can say you want to get a taste of a different approach. Don't hurt anyone's feelings or imply you aren't learning. I can assure you if you are with an expert NP, you are learning. You just might not be able to put all the pieces together yet. Orienting with a competent NP, someone who has been in role for more than 1 year, will be a completely different experience that you may better appreciate.

# Imposter Syndrome

Ahh, the imposter syndrome… Remember when you were first an RN and they took you off orientation kicking and screaming? You weren't ready, you needed more time! But they kicked you off anyway and you learned your role. You are in the same position now. There is only so much orientation can do for you. You need to learn the rules, the basics and the people around you. Everything else will be learned through your experiences – and that takes time and effort.

From the point when you are kicked off orientation to the time you walk into your facility and you are not in a full sweat may seem like a lifetime but you will get there. In the meantime you may suffer from the imposter syndrome.

The imposter syndrome is not something new or relevant only to nurse practitioners, it is common and well-studied. It is a phenomenon whereby a person has an internal experience of not belonging or being good enough to belong.

Do not take this feeling lightly! It needs to be validated and acknowledged. You may feel like you are smart enough or good enough to be where you are. You may think that you got where you are based on luck or by fooling others. There may even be a sense that people are overestimating you and you don't belong. You can find innumerable reasons for negating any external evidence to the contrary that you don't belong.

My advice is to allow the feelings wash over you, but don't let them take over you. We all feel an enormous sense of responsibility in the role of the NP. Unless you fabricated your masters degree and national certification, no one rightly believes you are a fraud or you don't belong.

You are just going to have to come to some level of consensus that you had some role in success getting to the level where you are. You have to believe that being wrong or not knowing something does not equal failure or make you a fake. As a new grad you are on a steep learning curve. You have to acknowledge the knowledge deficit you have and recognize the effort you need to reduce the gap.

In the larger context of the world, nobody really knows what they're doing, which can be both comforting and discomforting. People are always learning, trying, failing, succeeding and starting all over again. Any stage that you are in has nothing to do with whether you belong or not.

Nursing in general has this complex of not belonging at the table for important decisions being made in healthcare. It's important to embrace the feeling of being an imposter and know we all feel it.

I have a PhD in Nursing, this does not mean I am anymore an expert than you are in chess or wine tasting, or working as an NP on a trauma service. We would have the same learning curve to overcome.

Though I imagine I know more than just about anyone about return to work patterns in patients aged 18-65 who suffered from a grade I subarachnoid hemorrhage 1 year post injury.

Do I belong in the faculty of a prestigious school or working as a Senior Manager for a major retail organization? Based on my knowledge expertise – NO! But I'm willing to work hard, learn what I need to know, acknowledge when I don't know something, embrace my imposter-ness and be resourceful in finding the answers I need. No one really expects much more.

# Defining The Role Of The NP

You will find as you are advancing through the stages of competency and becoming the subject matter expert that the role of the NP becomes increasingly less defined instead of more defined. I see this as a huge positive! This opening, if you will, allows NPs today to pioneer roles that may not yet exist.

When I first started out on the neurosurgery service, I only did discharges. The neurosurgeons did not know what else to do with me. The residents saw me as a dumping outlet of things they didn't want to do. I embraced this position because I began taking on bigger and bigger tasks. You have to build the foundation strong to keep going up.

As I became more proficient in the tasks I was given, I was simply given more opportunities. The neurosurgery residents would say, did you ever try this? Or do you know how to do that?

Why don't you come down to the OR for a bit, etc. I just kept adding on skills. It's like when you learned about compounded interest in school. Saving a little bit of money in the short run might seem pointless, but as the little change adds up quickly it starts compounding at higher rates even faster.

The same will be true with your knowledge and skill set as a new NP. You don't have to learn one thing at a time. You should be learning many things simultaneously. It will take a bit longer, but you will better for it. When you become competent in one area, either focus on areas that are not as strong, or start looking for knowledge and skills that will complement what you do.

Don't stop with medical knowledge. Get involved in parts of your facility that interest you. You might want to become a subject matter expert in billing and coding or interpreting radiology or designing courses for new NPs! All of these skills will require you continue learning new topics and new subject matter.

**The goal as far as I am concerned is to never define the role of the NP.**

I want to watch it expand to infinity and beyond! From working in neurosurgery to academics to corporate America to the virtual space, I want keep pushing the limits. I would encourage you to do the same!!

# Why NPs Fail At Their First Job

There are several reasons why NPs fail at their first job. The number 1 reason in my opinion is simply an incompatible match between the new NP and the employer. Other reasons are lack of training and mentorship, destructive thinking, lack of interest and low productivity and a lack of persistence. Ok so let's break this down a bit.

## Incompatible Match

Many NPs when they graduate are overwhelmed by the number of opportunities that exist. Because the job market is so tight, NPs are being heavily recruited by hospitals, offices, insurance companies, healthcare agencies and beyond. If you haven't done your due diligence to try and figure out what your NP personality is and what kind of career lifestyle you are looking for, you may easily be enticed by opportunities that may not be right for you. All employers will put their best foot forward during the interview (just like you!) and you may be intimidated to press on certain areas that are important to know about your daily work when everyone is so nice!

It is so important for you to see the interview process as your time to get to know the employer. So many new NPs think this will be the only opportunity for an NP job and psych themselves out about being liked by the employer. When you interview, it is the only real opportunity you get to see if they are compatible with you, so make sure you make the best of it. You will also come off more confident if you believe you are interviewing them and not vice-versa. I don't mean for you to take this to extremes and be obnoxious. This should take the edge off of performing at the interview. The fact of the matter is you have the upper hand at this stage.

If you haven't done your self-assessment and you take a job that isn't compatible with your lifestyle or work style, it simply isn't going to work out. Don't talk yourself into a job that doesn't feel right.

# Lack Of Training

As you start your new job, you will need an orientation process that provides you basic knowledge of your subject area, how the facility runs, and how to get things done. Most facilities are pretty good about getting this information to you, but the delivery of it can be overwhelming. Imagine getting a stack of 50 seminal articles to read.

It's like being back in school – where do you start? What is essential to know? How do you translate reading into practice? It is very difficult to read an article and apply it to practice. You have to build upon a foundation of knowledge that starts with a very broad, simplistic overview. Then you can start deepening the knowledge. Providing all the knowledge you need at one time is a recipe for failure particularly if the only follow up is to grill you for answers to pop quiz questions.

# Lack Of Mentorship

We talked about this earlier in this book. Mentorship comes in many different forms from many different people. There isn't just one person who will mentor you in all areas of your life. You need to find mentors to help you with various milestones.

Some mentors can help you achieve multiple levels of milestones while some mentors can only help you achieve one milestone. You may think you want the expert NP at the facility to mentor you, but this could be a fatal mistake.

Expert NPs may not remember how they attained their knowledge milestones and may get frustrated by the new NP who just doesn't "get it". Expert NPs always seem to "know" what to do, but may not be able to explain it to a new NP. If you are orienting with an Expert NP but not doing well during orientation, this could be the problem.

The expert NP may simply be too smart and too good to teach. Remember this phenomenon in school?

The professor who was too smart to teach? Teaching something new requires someone who can break down the pieces so they are manageable. You don' t want Albert Einstein teaching you the theory of relativity the first time you hear it. You won't be ready for Einstein until you are in the advanced stages of understanding. The same is true with learning from your mentors.

It may be great to have a high level overview of your career from an expert, but don't expect that person to show you the blueprint of how to get there. You will need different mentors for that.

If you are struggling to understand your role and the basic knowledge to perform your job, consider whether you and your preceptor are a good match or not.

# Destructive Thinking

This could also be termed as self-sabotage. You are the type of person who needs to be the expert from the get-go and can't handle being a novice at something again. When you make mistakes, you are convinced that you are no-good and don't belong in the role of the NP.

Or you think everyone doesn't like you or think you are any good. All of these thoughts are destructive and self-filling. When you think negatively, you project negatively, so then people respond to you negatively, which reinforces your negative perceptions. It's a vicious cycle. The fact of the matter is, being a new NP is hard, humiliating and humbling.

You have to learn an entirely new skill set, you are publicly exposed as a novice and you realize you don't know nearly as much as you thought and only a fraction of what you should.

This is a huge learning curve, regardless of whichever specialty you choose to go into. You need to map out your milestones and create a plan to achieve them. Talk to your peers to make sure you are on target with where you should be and forgive yourself. This doesn't mean to dismiss a knowledge deficit. When you find a knowledge deficit, instead of berating yourself, write down some notes about what you need to know and follow up on it.

If you are destructive in your thinking, this will come out in your practice, which will lead other people to believe you don't know what you are doing, which leads them not to trust you. When I was a new NP, I said "I don't know" very frequently, but I always followed up on the answer. If you tell a colleague, a nurse, a patient or family member you don't know the answer, that is ok. But make sure you come back with one. This will not only gain their respect, but it will help you learn and detract from the destructive self-berating thoughts.

## Lack Of Interest And Low Productivity

I think these two attributes go hand in hand. If you don't like what you are doing, you aren't going to be interested or productive. This is the secret recipe of failing at your job. If the job or even the role of the NP isn't for you, then I would encourage you to find something else that is right for you. Most people want to feel like they are contributing to their career and their work. If you aren't inspired and excited about what you are doing, keep looking.

# Lack Of Persistence

There is nothing easy about becoming an NP, but it's fun and rewarding, so worth the effort! The last point I want to make mention on as a reason for failing in a job is a lack of persistence.

If something is worth having, it's worth working towards.

You will have great days and terrible days and every type of day in between. But at the end of the day you have to evaluate what you learned and what you need to learn. You have to be persistent in trying and trying again. You have to keep asking the same questions from different angles to really understand. Be persistent in your learning, be persistent in your understanding, be persistent in getting the knowledge you need and the mentorship to guide you through it all.

# Importance Of Mentorship

The importance of mentorship can't be overstated. This is evident now more than ever with the explosion of leadership courses, group and individual coaching, mentorship programs, etc. It is so important that most facilities now mandate some sort of mentorship to new employees.

However, mandated mentorship isn't exactly the most effective system. When I first started my job as nursing faculty, I was given a mandated mentorship with a person who was less than thrilled to be my "mentor". The person I was assigned to had been there for many years and knew how to get things done, but she was miserable! In fact, a year after I joined, she left. So how much mentoring do you think I got from this person?

Well, in fact, I got none. So I looked outside the institution and found the AANP mentorship program, which I applied to and was accepted into. This was a group program to help nurse practitioners with mounting a project of sorts. In the years following, I would have many different mentors in multiple different forms to help me with various projects. Most of my mentors have been at a distance (as you can't always have your teachers living in the same town!). My mentors live in Toronto, San Diego and Australia at the moment, so our virtual platform is the only media that works.

In your role as a new NP, you will need a couple different mentors as well. You will need to find someone at your facility who can help you navigate the system. This person does not need to be an NP, it may very well be the admin at the desk or the medical assistant who has been around for years.

But find someone to help you with basic issues. The next mentor needs to be a subject matter expert who can help you piece together a plan to address your knowledge deficit. This may very well be the NP preceptor or an MD, a resident, or a physician assistant. And finally you need someone who can help you see the bigger picture of what is going on, how to navigate the first several months and how to set your career on the right course.

I would encourage you to find someone who will have a vested interest in your career and who is able to help you map out your blueprint for success.

## Seeing The Big Picture

There is the big picture of where NPs fall into the healthcare system and then there is the microcosm in which you work and everything in between. In your first job, you will be laser focused on understanding your microcosm of a space, but it's important to understand that bigger picture as well.

However, to get started, I would strongly recommend you join the American Association of Nurse Practitioners. If you can only join one membership, please make it AANP. This group is only as powerful as we make it collectively. To date almost half the nation has independent practice for NPs thanks to the collaborative effort of AANP and the support of its members. As a new NP, you may not appreciate the meaning of full practice authority for NPs, but this is a huge win for us as a profession.

**AANP will give you that bigger picture you need to understand the full scope of the role of the NP.**

Be a part of it!

And full practice authority opens up the door to NursePreneurship, which I hope you will consider in a couple years when you are ready to move forward in your career.

We need NP Leaders, NursePreneurs and NP Change Agents. In essence, we need you to be ambitious in your career and you aspirations.

We need more NP Leaders out there. As once famously said: **If you aren't at the table you are on the menu!**

Healthcare is constantly changing and reforming with or without us. The more NPs who are out there advocating for best practice and access to care, the better. It really is everyone's obligation to move the NP profession forward.

Don't think you are a leader? Guess what most people don't either. Leadership is a learned skill. You will never be a leader unless you study it, work at it and apply it. So here is your first crash course in Leadership. It is never too early to learn basic leadership skills and it will open doors for you wherever you go.

Remember you will never be 100% ready for anything, but as Sir Richard Branson famously states:

*"If somebody offers you an amazing opportunity but you are not sure you can do it, say yes – then learn how to do it later!"*

You are just starting out, your colleagues will be very forgiving and will wait for you to reach your milestones. In the meantime get started on the right foot with the right people in your ballpark.

**Good Luck on starting your NP Career!!**

*Catie is a Nurse Practitioner, academic leader, entrepreneur, and proud mom. She has written, lectured and taught on many topics on advanced practice nursing, NP issues, post-graduate fellowships and mentoring. She is the founder of NursePreneurs, a website dedicated to sharing the amazing, exciting and inspiring work of NursePreneurs across the country.*

# ABOUT THE AUTHOR

Catie Harris, PhD, MBA and Registered Nurse is the NursePreneur Mentor who has empowered hundreds of nurses to monetize their knowledge and skills in business, while inspiring them to change the way healthcare is perceived and delivered. She strives to undo the perception that nursing care is limited to the hospital setting. Through her intensive mentorship program, Catie shows nurses how their nursing knowledge can transcend the hospital system into a profitable business.

Catie has been a nurse practitioner for over 10 years, and she has worked in corporate, academic and clinical settings. She owns The NP Life, Concierge Nurse Services, Hydration Operation and she is the host The NursePreneur Podcast.

Find out more and get free gifts and training at:

www.CatieHarris.com

Made in the USA
Coppell, TX
09 November 2022

86069545R00053